METABOLIC DIET

Beginner's Guide to a Metabolic Diet

Sam Lucky

Table of Contents

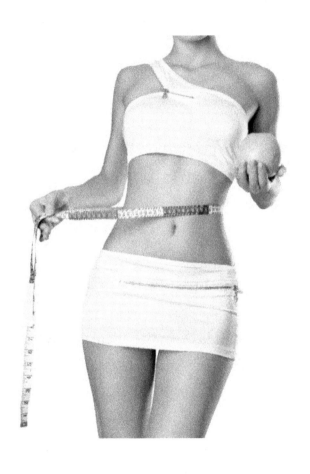

Introduction

**Eat more and weigh less? A diet with no
yo-yo effect when returning to a normal
calorie regimen?
This is exactly what the metabolic reset
promises!
Let's see in detail how it works.**

Metabolic reset is becoming increasingly
popular in the fitness industry and among
celebrities. The basic idea of the "reverse diet"
is weight maintenance during a normal calorie
regimen, both after a low-calorie diet and in
daily life. The result is a body in top shape.

Unfortunately, there are currently very few significant studies on metabolic reset, however this principle follows a very clear logic and the positive experiences reported by its fans are very promising.

Regardless of the diet we follow and what we prefer to eat, food should taste good and satisfy our tastes. Always! To reach or maintain a healthy weight, it is essential to choose the right foods.

What is a metabolic reset?

There are **two different definitions of a metabolic reset**. We'll explain both but delve primarily into the second, which involves a gradual increase in daily calories.

Metabolic reset: turn your habits upside down

One definition of a metabolic reset, or reverse diet, is eating **dinner in the morning, lunch in the middle of the day and breakfast in the evening.** The principle is simple: consume most of your calories in the morning and in the middle of the day because, thanks to the activities carried out in daily life, the body has plenty of time to burn them. The night, on the other hand, concentrates on regeneration and rest, without having to use the energy for digestion.

A good portion of carbohydrates, good fats and protein should speed up your metabolism in the morning and provide the boost you need for the day. Lunch should include a light meal with protein and fiber, and dinner should include a breakfast such as a yogurt and granola bowl, a smoothie bowl or an egg.

It takes getting used to, but this method can be really effective. At the end of the day, the important thing is always the **total calories, the** right distribution of carbohydrates, proteins, fats and the **choice of foods**: junk food and excess calories will not allow you to reach your goals, not even eating dinner at breakfast!

Metabolic reset: speed up your metabolism instead of starving yourself

The definition of reverse diet as "**diet after diet**" is clearly much more promising, but also more complex: you have to increase your daily caloric intake in a controlled way to speed up your metabolism, and once the metabolic reset is over, you can return to your normal caloric needs. In this way, after a diet it is easier to avoid the yo-yo effect and reactivate your sluggish metabolism.

This principle is based on the fact that if during a restrictive diet you constantly take in fewer calories than you consume, your body burns less and less of them and your metabolism goes into **energy-saving mode.** The body reacts in this way to **restore homeostasis**, i.e. to maintain the balance between physiological processes.

If **after finishing a diet** you suddenly increase your energy intake, **your body stores these unexpected calories as fat** and prepares itself for when you are hungry again. In this case the yo-yo effect occurs and in the worst case you can gain more weight than you lost.

This is where the metabolic reset comes into play: a slow, controlled increase in daily caloric intake allows the metabolism to be reactivated and accelerated, and also promotes an increase in diet-induced thermogenesis. Instead of forming fat pads, the body burns the calories taken in.

By eating more we are automatically less hungry, consequently we are happier and **we also produce less leptin**, the **hunger hormone** that slows down the metabolism and promotes the formation of fat pads useful for storing energy.

So far the theory is only confirmed by experience, in fact **currently there are no studies able to prove the effects of the reverse diet**. Nevertheless, we think it's worth a try!

Tip: Metabolic reset requires an accurate calculation of calories, but with our recipes you don't need to do that, we've taken care of it for you! Choose from more than 300 tasty ideas, obviously perfectly in line with your goals.

Here's how the metabolic reset works: 5 tips

For the metabolic reset to be effective, you need to follow some rules. Although we don't have scientific information about the reverse diet, we have enough **established dietary knowledge** that will help you increase your chances of success with the reverse diet.

#1 Increase calories, but slowly

In order to gradually awaken the metabolism, you need to be patient: as a rule, the caloric increase should be **50-100 kcal per week**.

Example:

If during the diet you took in about 1800 kcal daily, in the first week of the metabolic reset your daily caloric intake should be 1850-1900, in the second week go to 1900-1950 kcal, and so on. You must continue this way until you have figured out what is the daily caloric requirement that you can sustain without gaining weight.

The duration of the reverse diet depends on your deficit and your normal daily energy intake.

#2 Choose healthy foods

If you think you can increase your calories by eating candy bars, we must disappoint you. Your eating plan should include healthier foods with a low **glycemic index**, such as white yogurt, green lentils, whole grain rye bread, carrots, apples and cashews. This way the **insulin level** rises slowly and both **hunger attacks** and unnecessary storage of calories in the form of fat pads are avoided.

#3 Pay attention to macronutrients

If you've been following a good low-calorie diet, you've certainly calculated your **macronutrient needs.** Unless you radically change your lifestyle or the frequency with which you exercise, the percentage distribution of macronutrients may remain the same, especially during the first few weeks.

We suggest using our **free macronutrient calculator** every two weeks or so to make sure your current distribution is still in line with your goal and physical activity level.

The percentage of fat mass tells you if you are on track, so we suggest you calculate it at the beginning of the metabolic reset and check it every two weeks. If it grows more than 1%, review the amount of calories and the distribution of macronutrients. To remedy this quickly, increase your protein intake as little as possible, then reduce the percentage of carbohydrates to a minimum and stop increasing daily calories for a week.

If during the diet you have significantly increased the amount of protein intake, towards the middle of the metabolic reset begin to consume less by gradually introducing more carbohydrates.

#4 Practice physical activity

Have you been training to lose weight or to develop or define muscles? Then continue with that. However, if you change the duration of the training stimulus, your caloric needs will also change, whether you do more or less sport. Metabolic resetting requires great precision, so if you decide to try it, make sure you keep track of your training program. To do this, **fitness trackers** that help you determine your actual calorie consumption are very useful.

#5 Keep an overview

In order for the gradual increase in calories and the whole concept of diet after diet to be effective, it is essential to **pay attention to nutrition and physical activity**. The following points are particularly important:

- **The amount of calories taken in at the end of the diet.**
  How high was your caloric deficit or how many calories were you taking in daily before you started the metabolic reset? This information is critical in planning

your eating program. Write down the amount of calories you initially took in and consider a weekly increase of 50-100 calories. This way you can accurately calculate the number of weeks it will take to reach your goal.

- **How much do you eat?**
Keep track of every single calorie, even those in your apple juice or latte. Surpassing 50-100 kcal is much easier than you think, just consider that an average sized apple contains 50 kcal.

- **How much do you consume?**
There can be an abysmal difference between your calculated and actual calorie consumption, so you need to check it daily.

- **How much do you weigh?**
  Check your weight every day to avoid
  falling back into old patterns without
  realizing it, but don't worry too much if
  you have 1 kg too much every now and
  then. Full glycogen stores or water
  retention, especially in women due to
  their cycle, can affect weight, so
  fluctuations of 1-2 kg are very normal in
  both men and women. Before you get
  started, find out **how to weigh
  yourself correctly**.

Based on this information you can check at any
time if you have reached your daily goal and
where **you are in your journey**. After 3-4
weeks you will see that your metabolism will
react well to the increase in calories and you

will understand how long you should continue with the reverse diet.

Does this sound like a lot of work? Indeed it is, but it is definitely worth it to be able to **maintain the fitness you have achieved** and eat as you like.

Is metabolic reset healthy?

There is currently **no scientific knowledge** about the effects of the reverse diet on health, but just as with other dietary regimens, what you eat is crucial: choose **good fats**, **complex carbohydrates**, **quality proteins** and **fiber-rich foods**.

Eat more or less the same amount of food every day, distribute meals in a balanced way to **avoid insulin spikes** and make sure to keep your blood sugar stable. In this way you don't suffer from hunger attacks and you promote lipid metabolism.

Tip: You'll find **more than 300 healthy fitness recipes in** our free cookbook, and each one lists the exact amount of calories, protein and carbs it contains. They're perfect for reaching your goal and succeeding with the metabolic reset.

Who is the metabolic reset suitable for?

The reverse diet is suitable for all those who want to normalize their lifestyle and **avoid the**

yo-yo effect after following a low-calorie diet plan. It can also be effective if during a diet **you are unable to lose weight despite the caloric deficit**, in fact it helps to reactivate the metabolism and lose weight.

Following a muscle definition phase or after following a specific diet before a competition, the reverse diet is ideal to return to a normal caloric regimen without gaining too much weight.

Basically, the best thing to do is to write down and keep track of all the calories taken in. This procedure requires a lot of precision, which is why you need to invest a lot of time and energy in the diet to be followed after the diet.

Is tracking calories a must?

Constantly noting calories is necessary during metabolic resets and restrictive diets, but it can become an obligation. **Nutrition** is important to **achieve your goals, however it must also be enjoyable and healthy** for both body and soul.

Accurately documenting your macros and micronutrients over a period of time can certainly help you develop **a better relationship with food**, but it can also have the opposite effect.

It's possible that you may lose your body perception and taste for eating: if the idea of having to write down calories and sugar ruins your enjoyment of the occasional ice cream, you've reached a critical point. That's why we suggest you always keep an eye on your reactions.

In short

- Metabolic reset involves a gradual increase in calories after following a low-calorie diet.

- It helps avoid the yo-yo effect and is the first step in adopting healthier eating habits.

- It can be a measure to take if weight stalls during a diet.

METABOLIC DIET

- It requires you to record your caloric intake and consumption for a long time and accurately, leading to the risk of developing an unhealthy relationship with food, sport and your body.

- To date, there have been no representative studies of metabolic reset.

METABOLIC DIET

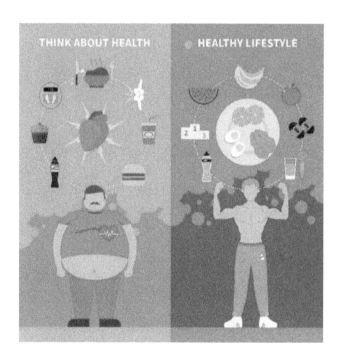

RECIPES

AIR "FRIED" CAULIFLOWER

INGREDIENTS
- 2 C fresh cauliflower florets
- 4 teaspoons oil (Roasted Garlic, Luscious Lemon, Valencia Orange or oil of your choice)
- 1 teaspoon Seasoning of your choice
- 1 pinch Dash of Desperation Seasoning

DIRECTION
Add the cauliflower to a large bowl.

Drizzle with oil and sprinkle with seasoning or glaze of your choice. Do NOT wash the bowl, simply set it aside.

Add to your air fryer basket in one layer. Careful not to overcrowd the basket- the air needs to circulate around each piece to crisp.

Cook on 400 for 4 minutes. Open the air fryer and toss the cauliflower. Cook for an additional 4 minutes.

Pour the cauliflower back into the bowl with the residual oil and seasoning. Sprinkle with a pinch of

Dash of Desperation (or salt and pepper) and toss to coat.
Serve hot.
Enjoy!

- Serving Size: 1/2 C cauliflower and is 0 Lean, 1 Green, 1 Healthy Fat and 2 Condiment options.

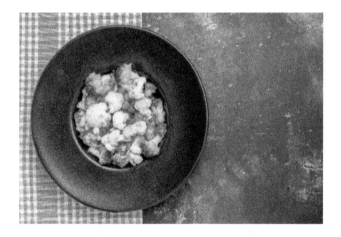

MEDITERRANEAN PORK LOIN WITH SUN DRIED
TOMATOES AND OLIVES

INGREDIENTS
- 11/2-2 lbs pork tenderloin (NOT marinated)
- 1 C Broth of your choice (chicken, vegetable, etc.)
- 2 teaspoons   Garlic and Spring Onion Seasoning or Garlic Gusto Seasoning (or Garlic, chives, lemon, salt, pepper, onion and garlic powder)
- 1/2 teaspoon   Mediterranean Seasoning
- 10 green olives, sliced
- 1 T sun dried tomatoes (not in oil) sliced thin

DIRECTION
Place pork loin in the bottom of the Crock Pot (slow cooker.)
Pour the broth over the meat.
Sprinkle with the seasonings, then scatter the olives and sun dried tomatoes around the meat.
Place the lid on and cook on high for 4 hours, or low for 6 hours. Meat may need longer if frozen. It will be done when the internal temperature reaches 155 degrees F.

Slice the meat thin, drizzle with some of the broth and garnish with a few olive and sun dried tomato pieces.
Serve hot.

- Serving Size: 5 ounces of pork tenderloin drizzled with 2 T of broth and is 1 Lean, 0 Green, 2 Condiments, 0 Healthy Fat

CREAMY SPINACH AND GARLIC STUFFED CHICKEN

INGREDIENTS
- 1 1/2 lbs boneless, skinless chicken breast
- 8 T (1/2 of an 8 oz block) light cream cheese
- 1 Tablespoon Garlic and Spring Onion Seasoning or Garlic Gusto Seasoning (or Garlic, chives, lemon, salt, pepper, onion and garlic powder)
- 8 ounces raw baby spinach (1 bag)
- 1 pinch Dash of Desperation Seasoning

DIRECTION
Preheat oven to 375 degrees.

Place chicken breast on a cutting board and using a sharp knife, cut a pocket into the chicken breast. Repeat on all pieces of chicken.

Place the cream cheese into a large microwave safe bowl and heat on high for 10 seconds until soft and spreadable. Repeat in 5 second intervals if necessary. Sprinkle the garlic seasoning over the cream cheese. Stir to combine & smooth out all the lumps.

Pour the spinach into the bowl. Using a pair of kitchen shears, chop up the spinach into smaller pieces.

Using a rubber spatula, combine the spinach and the cream cheese together into a consistent mixture. Do this gently as to not crush and bruise the spinach.

Divide the mixture into as many equal portions as you have pieces of chicken. Stuff mixture into the pocket of the chicken breast. Repeat on all pieces of chicken.

Place chicken in an oven safe dish side by side. Use a dish that is large enough to leave space around each piece so they are not touching. (This allows for faster, more even cooking.)

Using a rubber spatula, get the remaining cream cheese out of the bowl and place a little smear on top of each of the chicken rolls to protect them while baking. Sprinkle each with a pinch of Dash of Desperation seasoning. You can also spray with a little nonstick cooking spray if there doesn't seem to be "enough" cream cheese left.

Cover the dish with aluminum foil and place in the center of your preheated oven.

Bake for 35 minutes, remove the foil and bake for an additional 10 minutes or until chicken has reached an internal temperature of 165 degrees as verified with a meat thermometer.

Let chicken rest for 5 minutes and then slice and serve.

- Serving Size: 8.7 ounces of cooked Creamy Spinach and Garlic Stuffed Chicken and is 1 Lean, .5 Green, 3 Condiments, 0 Healthy Fat

CHEESY CHICKEN & CAULIFLOWER BAKE

INGREDIENTS

- 1 1/2 pounds boneless, skinless chicken breasts cut into 3/4" chunks
- 2 teaspoons Roasted Garlic Oil (or Garlic and oil of your choice)

- pinch Dash of Desperation Seasoning (or Garlic, onion, salt, pepper, parsley)
- 6 T Half and Half
- 1 Garlic and Spring Onion Seasoning (or Garlic, chives, natural sea salt, onion and garlic powder)
- 6 cups grated cauliflower (fresh works best, but you can also use frozen)
- 1 C light OR 1/2 C regular shredded cheddar cheese

DIRECTION
Preheat oven to 325 degrees.
In a large skillet, heat Roasted Garlic Oil over medium-high heat.
Add the chicken to the skillet, season with a pinch of Dash of Desperation and saute until slightly golden brown and tender (about 10-12 minutes.)
While chicken is cooking, cut the cauliflower into smaller pieces and grate into "rice" using a box grater into a large bowl. You may also do this by pulsing a few pieces at a time in the food processor
Spray a 9x11 baking dish with nonstick cooking spray and add the cauliflower into a single layer in the bottom of the dish.
Sprinkle the chicken in the skillet with Garlic and Spring Onion Seasoning. Pour the half and half into

the skillet and stir, scraping up all the browned bits off the bottom.

Pour the chicken and cream mixture over the cauliflower and sprinkle with the cheese.

Cover tightly with aluminum foil and bake for 15-20 minutes until hot and melty.

Serve hot and enjoy!

- Serving Size: 1/4 of this dish (approximately 1 1/2 C Cauliflower and 6 ounces chicken breast) and is 1 Leaner, 3 Green, 3 Condiments, 1 Healthy Fat. Nutrition information is calculated using regular, not low fat cheddar cheese

FINGER LICKING SLOW COOKED BBQ CHICKEN

INGREDIENTS

- 2 pounds boneless, skinless chicken thighs
- 1 Honey BBQ Seasoning (or a dry, sugar free substitute)
- 1 Tablespoon of Phoenix Sunrise or Southwestern Seasoning (or cumin, cayenne, chili powder, salt, pepper, garlic and onion)
- pinch Alderwood Smoked Sea Salt (or)

DIRECTION

Place chicken thighs in a single layer at the bottom of your slow cooker. (You could use an Insta Pot as well, 10 minutes cooking time)

Sprinkle seasonings over the thighs. Place the cover on the slow cooker.

Cook on low for 6 hours.

Remove the lid and using two forks, shred the meat. Serve hot with your favorite side dishes, or chilled over a salad.

- Serving Size: 5 ounces of chicken is 1 Lean and 2 Condiment options.

SKEWERED SHRIMP WITH LEEKS AND YELLOW SQUASH

INGREDIENTS
- 2 pounds wild caught shrimp, raw, peeled & deveined
- 2 large leeks, washed, trimmed and cut into 1/2" chunks
- 2 small, thinner yellow squash, washed, trimmed and cut into 1/2" chunks
- 1 Tablespoon of Rockin' Ranch (or tarragon, chives, garlic, lemon, salt, pepper, garlic and onion)
- 2 1/2 Tablespoons Luscious Lemon or Roasted Garlic Oil
- 8 T fresh grated Parmesan cheese for garnish
- Natural Sea salt & fresh cracked peppercorns (or a pinch of Dash of Desperation) to taste

DIRECTION
Preheat outdoor grill or oven to 375 degrees.
Add the shrimp and veggies to a large bowl. Drizzle with oil and seasonings. Toss to coat. Let sit for 10

minutes, up to all day (refrigerated) to let the flavors develop.

Skewer shrimp and veggies individually, or pour into a grill basket.

Cook for 20-25 minutes, using a spatula to turn the pieces at least once during cooking. Cook until shrimp is opaque and fully cooked and vegetables are crisp-tender.

Serve hot, sprinkled with fresh grated Parmesan cheese for a garnish,

- Serving Size: Because of the mixed nature of this dish, to portion go by weight. 14.5 ounces of shrimp, mixed veggies & 1 Tablespoon Parmesan Cheese is 1 Leanest, 3 Green, 3 Condiments and 2 Healthy Fat

MOJO MARINATED FLANK STEAK

INGREDIENTS

- 2 pounds flank steak or skirt steak, trimmed of all excess fat
- 2 fresh lime juice plus 1 extra lime for garnish
- 1 Garlic and Spring Onion (or fresh garlic, onion, chives, parsley, salt, pepper)
- 1 tsp ground cumin (optional, but will give more flavor)
- 1/3 C low sodium beef broth
- 1 pinch   Dash of Desperation Seasoning

DIRECTION

Add all ingredients (except beef & Dash) to a large zipper style bag. Zip closed & using your hands, smoosh all the ingredients together to make a uniform marinade.

Add the beef. Seal again and place on a plate, in the refrigerator for 1 hour up to overnight.

When ready to cook, preheat outdoor grill (or indoor cast iron pan or grill pan) to medium high heat. Oil the grates or the pan lightly using nonstick cooking spray prior to heating.

Remove the steak from the bag and discard the marinade. Season with the Dash of Desperation.

Cook the steak for 2 minutes on each side and check the temperature. Keep cooking / flipping until the internal temperature of the steak is 115-120 degrees for Medium Rare, 125-130 for Medium.

When finished cooking, remove from the pan and set on a plate. Tent the beef with foil and let it rest for 10 minutes. Finish your other sides during this time.

Slice the steak on a diagonal, garnish with lime wedges and serve hot with your favorite Green sides.

Enjoy!

- Serving Size: 5 oz. sliced beef and is 1 Lean, 0 Green, 0 Healthy Fat and 1 Condiment options. The marinade only imparts flavor to the steak and is discarded after use and does not need to be counted as it is not consumed.

CREAMY ASPARAGUS AND CHICKEN ROULADE

INGREDIENTS

- 1 1/2 lbs boneless, skinless chicken breast
- 8 T (1/2 of an 8 oz block) light cream cheese
- 1 Tablespoon Garlic and Spring Onion Seasoning (or Garlic, chives, lemon, salt, pepper, onion and garlic powder)
- 10 ounces raw asparagus (weighed after trimming ends)
- 1 pinch Dash of Desperation Seasoning

DIRECTION

Preheat oven to 375 degrees.

Place chicken breast in a large zipper bag on a sturdy cutting board. (NOT directly on the counter- they can crack!) Using the back of a medium sized, heavy frying pan, hit the meat holding the pan flat and pound it until 1/4" thin.* Repeat until all pieces are thin.

Place the cream cheese in a microwave safe bowl and heat on high for 10 seconds until soft and spreadable. Repeat in 5 second intervals if necessary. Stir to smooth out all the lumps.

Spread the cream cheese evenly over one side of all the chicken pieces and then sprinkle with Garlic & Spring Onion Seasoning.

Line the asparagus up on the chicken, leaving 1/2" free at each end.

Starting at one end, gently roll the chicken up into a "log" and place seam side down in a baking dish. Repeat the process until all the chicken and asparagus are used. (Note- do leave about a Tablespoon of cream cheese unused as we'll need that for the end)

Using a rubber spatula, get the remaining cream cheese out of the bowl and place a little smear on top of each of the chicken rolls to protect them while baking. Sprinkle each with a pinch of Dash of Desperation seasoning.

Cover the dish with aluminum foil and place in the center of your preheated oven.10.   Bake for 35 minutes, remove the foil and bake for an additional 10 minutes or until chicken has reached an internal temperature of 165 degrees.

Let chicken rest for 5 minutes and then slice and serve.

* If the chicken breasts are particularly thick, cut them in half through the middle before pounding. The best way to do this is to put the meat on the board, place your palm flat over the chicken to hold it still and carefully, with your knife blade parallel to the countertop, slice through the chicken.

- Serving Size: 8.5 ounces of cooked Creamy Asparagus and Chicken Roulade and is 1 Lean, 1 Green, 2 Condiments, 1 Healthy Fat

LOW-CARB CHICKEN SCARPARIELLO

INGREDIENTS
- 1 lb hot or sweet Italian style sausage (use turkey sausage for the leanest option)
- 1 lb boneless skinless chicken breast
- 5 C green peppers (about 5 medium) (Italain, bell, poblano, etc.) chopped into similar size pieces
- 1/4 of a medium onion, sliced (about .4 ounces)
- 1 Tablespoon   Garlic and Spring Onion Seasoning (or fresh garlic, onion, scallions, parsley, salt , pepper)
- 1/3 c low sodium chicken broth or water

DIRECTION
Slice the sausage into 1/2" thick slices (kitchen shears work great for this)

Chop the chicken and peppers into approximately equal size chunks.
Place a large frying pan with higher sides (see image below) on the stove over medium-high heat
Add the sausage and cook for 2 minutes, stirring occasionally.
Add the chicken, peppers and sprinkle with the Garlic Seasoning. Stir to combine./step]
Cook uncovered for 18-20 minutes, stirring frequently.
When finished, you should have a nice brown crust on the meat and a little in the bottom of the pan.
Turn the heat up to high and add the liquid. Scrape the bottom of the pan to release all the fond (brown yummy stuff) off the bottom of the pan.
Keep simmering until the liquid is reduced by half (should only be a minute or so) Remove from heat and serve hot.

- Serving Size: 6 oz. chicken/sausage and 1 C Vegetables and is 1 Leaner 3 Green, 1 Healthy Fat and 3 Condiment options.

PERFECT PAN SEARED TUNA

INGREDIENT
- 1 1/2 pounds of sushi quality tuna
- 4 teaspoons Valencia Orange Oil
- splash of low sodium soy
- squirt of wasabi paste
- 1 tablespoon of fresh ginger & 1 capful of Toasted Sesame Ginger Seasoning.

Enjoy!

- Serving: 7 ounces of fish (1 Lean) and 1 Tablespoon Sauce (2 condiments for the sauce & seasoning on fish) 1 teaspoon Valencia Orange Oil (1 Healthy Fat)

TUSCAN GETAWAY BAKED CHICKEN

INGREDIENTS
- 1 3/4 pounds boneless chicken thighs
- 1 Tablespoon Tuscan Fantasy Seasoning (or Garlic, Red pepper, black pepper, salt, onion, parsley, oregano, lemon, thyme and marjoram)

DIRECTION
Preheat oven to 375 degrees.
Place chicken in a baking dish large enough to hold all the pieces without touching.
Sprinkle seasoning over the meat equally.
Bake in the oven for 30-35 minutes until chicken reaches an internal temperature of 165 degrees.
Remove from heat and let rest on a plate for 5 minutes before serving.
- Serving Size: 5 ounces of cooked chicken and is 1 Lean, 0 Green, 1 Condiment, 0 Healthy Fat

TENDER ROSEMARY PORK LOIN

INGREDIENTS

- 1 1/2 pounds thin sliced (~1/2″) boneless, skinless pork loin, any and all excess fat trimmed**
- 1 Tablespoon Rosemary Versatility Seasoning (or Garlic, Rosemary, Sage, Thyme, Parsley, Onion, Black Pepper, Salt)
- 4 Teaspoons Roasted Garlic Oil (or Garlic, and oil of your choice)

DIRECTION

Preheat outdoor grill or indoor oven to 375 degrees. In a small bowl, combine oil and seasoning together to make a paste.

Pat the pork loin dry and slather equal amounts of seasoning on one side of each piece of meat.

Place the chops on the grill (or place in a baking dish and put in the oven) and cook until pork reaches 150 degrees. (Approximately 5-7 minutes on each side if using the grill, or 20-25 minutes in the oven.)

Remove from heat and let rest on a plate for 5 minutes before serving.

- Serving Size: 6 ounces of cooked pork and is 1 Leaner, 0 Green, 1 Condiments, 1 Healthy Fat

LOW CARB SHAKSHUKA

INGREDIENTS

- 1 pound bag riced cauliflower (frozen works great)
- 4 teaspoons good quality extra virgin olive oil
- 4 Tablespoons chopped onion
- 1 Tablespoon Spices of India Seasoning (or Garlic, ground mustard, turmeric, cumin, cayenne, natural sea salt, ground coriander)
- 1 15 ounce can diced tomatoes (no sugar added)
- 1 15 ounce can pureed tomatoes (no sugar added)
- 6 fresh eggs
- Fresh parsley for garnish if desired

DIRECTION

Cook cauliflower as perDIRECTIONs on package. (I microwaved a one pound bag that was frozen on high for 5 minutes & it was perfect)
Add the oil to a larger skillet (that has a lid) and heat over medium high heat.
Add the onions and saute for 1-2 minutes until translucent. /step]

Sprinkle the spices over the onions and oil and saute for 1 minute until fragrant.

Add the cauliflower to the skillet and stir to combine with the spices. Sprinkle with a little natural sea salt (if desired).

Add the tomatoes and stir to combine everything together.

Place the lid on the skillet and bring the dish to a boil. Let simmer for 5 minutes.

Remove the lid and gently crack the eggs over the tomato mixture. Season eggs with a pinch of salt and pepper (or Dash of Desperation for more flavor!) Put the lid on and let the eggs poach. 2-3 minutes for a poached egg with runny yolk, 5-7 minutes for an egg cooked hard. Sprinkle with fresh parsley as garnish if desired.

Remove from heat and enjoy!

- Serving Size: 1 1/2 C shakshuka mixture and 2 eggs and is 1 Lean, 3 Green, 3 Condiments, 1 Healthy Fat

PRIMAVERA MIXED GRILL

INGREDIENTS

- 1 3/4 lb boneless skinless chicken breast
- 7 C fresh vegetables, chopped into similar size pieces
- 4 tsp Roasted Garlic Oil (or oil of your choice)
- 1 Tablespoon Garlic Gusto Seasoning (or seasoning of your choice
- 1 Tablespoon Dash of Desperation Seasoning (or seasoning of your choice

DIRECTION

Preheat outdoor grill (or indoor oven) to 400 degrees.

Peel, seed and chop the vegetables into 1" chunks. Add to a large bowl.

Cut the chicken into 1" chunks. Add to the bowl.

Pour oil and seasonings over the chicken & veg and toss to coat.

Place mixture into a grill basket and place on the grill. (Or baking dish and into the oven)

Close the lid and cook for 30 minutes, tossing the mixture 1/2 way through cooking for even browning. Meal will be ready when chicken reaches 165 degrees (verify with a meat thermometer)

Remove from the heat and scoop the mixture into your favorite serving dish. Let the chicken rest for a few minutes before serving and enjoy!
Serve hot for dinner and any leftovers can be enjoyed chilled the next day.

- Serving Size: 6 oz. chicken and 1 1/2 C Vegetables and is 1 Leaner 3 Green, 1 Healthy Fat and 3 Condiment options.

CHEESY PEPPER TACO BAKE

INGREDIENTS
- 1lb 95-97% lean ground beef (chicken or turkey)
- 1 Phoenix Sunrise or Southwest Seasoning (or garlic, cumin, paprika, cayenne, salt, black pepper, onion and parsley)
- 1C no sugar added, fresh vegetable salsa plus 4 additional Tablespoons for garnish
- 1 1/2 lbs fresh peppers (green, red, poblano, your choice) stems removed, cut in half lengthwise and seeded.
- 1/2 C shredded lowfat cheddar cheese
- 4 T Sour Cream

DIRECTION

Preheat oven to 350 degrees.

Add ground meat, seasoning and salsa to a large bowl. Mix with your fingers to combine.

Divide the meat mixture equally among the pepper halves, loosely stuffing each. Place in the bottom of a large baking dish.

Sprinkle peppers with cheese.

Bake in preheated oven for 30 minutes, or until beef reaches 160 degrees F.

Remove from oven and divide into 4 equal servings. Top each serving with 1 T each of sour cream and salsa. Serve hot.

THAI CASHEW CHICKEN

INGREDIENTS

- 4 tsp Luscious Lemon Oil or Roasted Garlic Oil or oil of your choice
- 1 1/2 lbs boneless, skinless chicken breast cut into thin strips
- 1 T Tasty Thai Seasoning or garlic, onion, lemongrass, salt, red bell pepper, black pepper, lime zest and chiles
- 2 C green bell pepper, cut into thin strips

- 2 C red bell pepper, cut into thin strips
- 3 scallions sliced- separate whites and greens
- 24 cashews chopped into small pieces

DIRECTION

Heat oil in a large frying pan over medium high heat.

Add chicken to the pan and cook for 3-5 minutes on each side until opaque.

Add peppers and whites of scallions to the pan and sprinkle with seasoning. Stir to combine.

Cover and cook over high heat for an additional 5-7 minutes, stirring occasionally until vegetables are crisp tender and chicken is fully cooked.

Remove lid and sprinkle with nuts and scallion greens. Serve hot.

- Serving Size: 1/4 of this dish or, 6 ounces chicken and 1 Cup of vegetables and is 1 Leaner, 2 Green, 1 Healthy Fat and 3 Condiment options.

SUMMER SHRIMP PRIMAVERA

INGREDIENTS

- 4 teaspoons Luscious Lemon or Roasted Garlic Oil
- 2 pounds wild caught shrimp, raw, peeled & deveined
- 1 Tablespoon of Garlic and Spring Onion Seasoning or Simply Brilliant Seasoning (or sea salt, scallions, fresh garlic, lemon & parsley)
- 1/2 C low sodium chicken broth
- 6 C vegetable noodles
- 1 scallion, green tops only, sliced for garnish if desired
- 8 T fresh grated Parmesan cheese for garnish

DIRECTION

Make the vegetable noodles by spiralizing or using a vegetable peeler like I did to make big, wide noodles. Place noodles in a bowl and set aside.

Place the oil in the pan over medium-high heat and let it get hot.

Add the shrimp to the pan and cook for 3-4 minutes on one side before turning to cook on the other side. Sprinkle with seasoning and continue to cook for an additional 3 minutes. Add the broth to deglaze the pan and cook 1-2 minutes more, until shrimp are fully cooked.

Using a slotted spoon, remove the shrimp from the pan and set aside in a bowl.

Put the pan back over heat and heat until liquid is bubbling. Add the veggie noodles and saute for 1-2 minutes, until crisp-tender.

Add the veggie noodles to a serving bowl. Top with the shrimp and sprinkle with scallions and Parmesan cheese before serving.

Divide everything into 4 equal portions and serve hot.

- Serving Size:7 oz shrimp, 1.5 C veggie noodles and is 1 Lean, 3 Green, 2 Condiments and 2 Healthy Fat

OVEN ROASTED COD WITH POBLANO PEPPER GARLIC CREAM SAUCE

INGREDIENTS
- 5.5 ounces poblano peppers, seeded & sliced (2 Green)
- 1 C sour cream (8 Healthy Fat)
- 1 Tablespoon of Garlic and Spring Onion Seasoning (or sea salt, scallions, fresh garlic & parsley) (6 condiments)
- 5 C riced cauliflower, uncooked (10 Green)
- 1/4 C water
- 2 pounds flaky white fish, such as cod, flounder or halibut (4 Lean)

DIRECTION
Preheat oven to 375 degrees.

Place peppers, sour cream and seasoning into a food processor. Pulse until fully blended.

Add the cauliflower to the bottom of a 9x12 baking dish. Place the fish on top of the cauliflower in a single layer. Season with a little Salt & Pepper or a pinch of Dash of Desperation.

Dollop the pepper mixture over the fish equally, spreading evenly over the fish with the back of a spoon.

Pour the water into the cauliflower (pour in a corner of the dish as to not disturb the sauce.)
Bake for 25-35 minutes until fish is fully cooked, opaque and flaky. May take longer for fish over 1/2" thickness.
Divide everything into 4 equal portions and serve hot.

- Serving Size: 7 oz fish, 1/4 of the sauce, 1.5 C cauliflower rice and is 1 Lean, 3 Green, 1.5 Condiments and 2 Healthy Fat

CASHEW CHICKEN & CAULIFLOWER RICE

INGREDIENTS

- 4 tsp Valencia Orange Oil or unrefined coconut oil
- 3 scallions sliced into thin medallions
- 1 1/2 lbs boneless skinless chicken breast cut into thin strip
- 1 C green bell pepper cut into thin strips
- 1 C red bell pepper cut into thin strips
- 2 C additional vegetables of your choice (broccoli, snow peas, zucchini, etc.)

- 1 T Garlic Gusto, Garlic & Spring Onion, or Tasty Thai, Wok On or Simply Brilliant Seasoning (or fresh garlic, chives, salt, pepper, onion and parsley)
- 1/2 C low soduim chicken broth (if needed)
- 2 C prepared cauliflower rice
- 24 cashews, chopped into small pieces

DIRECTION

Add oil to a large frying pan over medium high heat. When hot, add scallion and cook for 1 minute until fragrant.

Add chicken and cook for 5-7 minutes until opaque. Add all the vegetables and sprinkle with seasoning. If you are using thicker, heavier vegetables like broccoli, add the broth to help steam/cook them a little faster. Cover with a lid and allow to cook for 5 more minutes until veggies are crisp-tender, but not overdone.

While chicken is cooking, prepare cauliflower rice. Remove chicken mixture from heat. Divide cauliflower rice into 4 equal portions. Do the same with the chicken mixture.

Place the chicken over the rice and sprinkle with 1/4 of the crushed cashews. Serve hot and enjoy!

- Serving Size: 6 oz. chicken breast and 1 1/2 C vegetables and is 1 Leaner, 3 Green, 1 Healthy Fat and 3 Condiment option.

Nutrition information below is calculated using only broccoli as the additional vegetable.

SWEET POTATO MUFFINS FUELING HACK

INGREDIENTS:
- 1 packet Honey Sweet potatoes
- 2 Tablespoon liquid egg (like Eggbeaters)
- 1/2 C water
- 1/4 tsp baking powder
- 2 pinches Awesome Autumn Seasoning or Sinful Cinnamon Seasoning

INSTRUCTION:
Preheat oven to 350 degrees (a toaster oven or the air fryer work great)
Mix first 4 ingredients and 1 pinch of Cinnamon together into a bowl.
Grease 2 muffin tins (or 2 small dishes about 1/2 C each) with nonstick cooking spray. Leftovers of the

little square baking "pans" that come with other Fuelings work well for this too.

Spoon equal amounts of the mixture into the 2 baking dishes.

Sprinkle with a pinch of cinnamon.

Bake for 15 minutes until thoroughly cooked. Verify with a toothpick (stick it in the middle and if it comes out clean, it's done.)

Enjoy warm!

- Counts: 2 Muffins is 1 Fueling and 1 Condiment (eggbeaters & seasoning)

GINGER LIME CHICKEN AND NOODLES

INGREDIENTS
- Hawkins Valencia 4 tsp Orange Oil
- 1 Tablespoon Tasty Thai Seasoning (or garlic, lemongrass, lime, ginger, orange zest, red pepper, onion, salt and pepper)
- juice of one lime
- 1 1/2 lbs boneless, skinless chicken breasts (cut in half if large)
- 4 C prepared zucchini noodles (here's an easy recipe for zoodles)

DIRECTION

Add first three ingredients to a large zipper style plastic bag.

Massage the plastic bag to combine the ingredients to make the marinade. Place chicken in the bag, squeeze out all the air, seal the bag and store in the refrigerator for 4 hours, up to overnight.

When ready to cook the chicken, preheat outdoor grill (or indoor grill pan or frying pan). Cook chicken on both sides for 12-15 minutes over medium high heat, until chicken is fully cooked. Verify temperature with meat thermometer.

While chicken is cooking, prepare zucchini noodles. (Here's an easy recipe for zoodles)

Serve chicken over zoodles, or with your favorite side dish and enjoy!

- Serving Size: 6 oz. chicken breast and 1 C zucchini noodles and is 1 Leaner, 2 Green, 1 Healthy Fat and 2 Condiment option.

CRISPY KHOLRABI SLAW

INGREDIENTS
- 4 C kohlrabi, sliced into matchsticks
- 1/4 C cilantro, chopped
- 1 teaspoons Phoenix Sunrise Seasoning (or your favorite no-salt taco style seasoning)
- 1 teaspoons Kickin' Cajun Seasoning* (or garlic, salt, black pepper, cumin, cayenne pepper and onion)
- Zest of 1 lime
- Zest of 1 orange
- Juice of 1 lime
- 4 teaspoons Valencia Orange Oil (or your favorite oil and fresh squeezed orange juice)

DIRECTION
Place all ingredients, except the kohlrabi & cilantro into a large salad bowl. Whisk to combine.
Add the kohlrabi to the bowl, sprinkle with cilantro. Using two large spoons, pull the dressing up through the salad by placing the spoons at the bottom of the bowl and scooping the kohlrabi mixture upward. Keep tossing until fully coated. Set aside for 15 minutes up to a day ahead of time and serve chilled.

- Serving Size: 1/2 C kohlrabi salad and is 0 Lean, 1 Green, 1/2 Healthy Fat and 1 Condiment options.

PAN SEARED PORK LOIN AND BALSAMIC CARAMELIZED ONIONS

INGREDIENTS
- nonstick cooking spray
- 1 teaspoons Dash of Desperation Seasoning (or garlic, salt, black pepper, onion and parsley)
- 1 1/2 lbs pork tenderloin (or beef tenderloin, or chicken breasts)

DIRECTION
Preheat oven (or outdoor BBQ Grill) to 400 degrees.
Season the tenderloin on both sides with Dash of Desperation Seasoning
Place a cast iron skillet (or oven-safe pan) on the stove over high heat. Spray with nonstick cooking spray.

When the pan is good and hot, place the tenderloins in the center, but try not to let them touch each other.
Cook tenderloin for 2-3 minutes on each side until browned.
Add the pork tenderloin back to the pan and place in the oven for 15-25 minutes until pork is fully cooked (larger pieces will take a bit longer). Verify temp with meat thermometer. Pork should be 145 degrees F to be slightly pink, 160 for medium. Take it out at desired temp and let rest for 3 minutes before slicing. Note- If pork is cooked more than these recommended temperatures, it will be very dry and overdone.
While the pork is roasting, whip up a batch of Balsamic Caramelized Onions.
Slice the pork and serve with Onions. Serve hot with your favorite side dish.

- Serving Size: 5 oz. pork with 2 T onions and is 1 Lean, 0 Green, 0 Healthy Fat and 1.5 Condiment options. Nutrition information below is for recipe made with pork tenderloin and onions inclusive.

BALSAMIC CARAMELIZED ONIONS

INGREDIENTS
- nonstick cooking spray
- 1 C onion slices
- 1/4 C low sodium chicken broth
- 4 Tablespoon Balsamic Mosto Cotto (or a balsamic reduction DO NOT use balsamic vinegar- it will be too tart)
- pinch of Dash of Desperation Seasoning (or sea salt and fresh cracked peppercorns)

DIRECTION
Place a medium sized frying pan on the stove over medium heat.
Add the onions and the broth and cook for 15-20 minutes, stirring occasionally. Try not to let the onions brown.
When onions are soft and liquid has evaporated, add the balsamic. Turn off heat, stir and let onions steep in the balsamic while pan remains on the stove.
Serve hot over grilled meats or chilled on salads.
May remain refrigerated for up to 1 week.

- Serving Size:2 Tablespoon of Onions and is equal to 1.5 Condiments.

CITRUS SHRIMP & SPINACH

INGREDIENTS

- 2 lbs wild caught, raw shrimp, cleaned and tails removed
- 4 tsp Luscious Lemon Oil
- 1 Tablespoon Simply Brilliant Seasoning (or garlic, lemon, onion, lemon and black pepper)
- 6 cups baby spinach greens, arugula greens, beet greens or a combination

DIRECTION

Heat oil in a large frying pan over medium high heat.

Add shrimp and sprinkle with seasoning. Stir to coat and cook 3-4 minutes, stirring occasionally. Shrimp should be opaque and cooked on both sides.

Add the greens to the pan. Using a pair of tongs, toss the greens in the pan for a minute or two until just wilted.

Serve hot.

- Serving Size: 7 oz. shrimp and 1 1/2 cups of greens and is 1 Leanest, 3 Green, 1 Healthy Fat and 1 Condiment option.

LEMON DILL ROASTED RADISHES

INGREDIENTS

- 4 C red radish halves, greens and stems removed
- 2 teaspoons high quality cooking oil of your choice
- 1/2 T Citrus Dill Seasoning
- 1/2 T Brightening Blend (or fresh squeezed lemon)

DIRECTION

Preheat oven to 350 degrees

Trim ends and tops of radishes, cut in half (all radish pieces should be about the same size- if you have small ones, leave them whole, big ones should be cut in 1/4, etc)

Add all ingredients to a large bowl and toss to coat. Place radishes in an oven-save roasting dish and place in oven, center rack, for 30 minutes. If you have a cast iron skillet, this is the PERFECT time to use it!

Serve hot

- Serves 4

MEDITERRANEAN ROASTED CHICKEN WITH LEMON DILL RADISHES

INGREDIENTS
- 2 lbs chicken thighs (If using bone-in chicken, add additional cooking time)
- Pinch Dash of Desperation Seasoning (or garlic, salt, black pepper, onion and parsley)
- 1 Tablespoon Mediterranean Seasoning (or garlic, marjoram, basil, rosemary and onion)

DIRECTION
Preheat oven (or outdoor BBQ Grill) to 375 degrees.
Season the chicken with just a pinch of Dash of Desperation Seasoning
Place the chicken in a baking dish large enough to hold them without touching one another (this speeds up the cooking process.)
Sprinkle chicken with Mediterranean seasoning.
Bake in preheated oven for 30 minutes, or until chicken reaches 165 degrees F.
Remove from oven and serve hot, or chilled over greens for salad.
- Serving Size: 5 oz. chicken and is 1 Lean, 0 Green, 0 Healthy Fat and 1 Condiment options. Nutrition

PORK TENDERLOINS AND MUSHROOMS

INGREDIENTS

- nonstick cooking spray
- 1 teaspoons Dash of Desperation Seasoning (or garlic, salt, black pepper, onion and parsley)
- 1 1/2 lbs pork tenderloin (or beef tenderloin, or chicken breasts)
- 6 cups portobello mushroom caps, cut into chunks
- 1/2 C low sodium chicken broth
- 1 Tablespoon Garlic Gusto or Garlic & Spring Onion Seasoning (or garlic, salt, black pepper, onion, paprika and parsley)
- fresh parsley for garnish if desired

DIRECTION

Preheat oven (or outdoor BBQ Grill) to 400 degrees.

Season the tenderloin on both sides with Dash of Desperation Seasoning

Place a cast iron skillet (or oven-safe pan) on the stove over high heat. Spray with nonstick cooking spray.

When the pan is good and hot, place the tenderloins in the center, but try not to let them touch each other.
Cook tenderloin for 2-3 minutes on each side until browned.
Remove the pork from the pan and set aside.
Leaving the pan on the heat, add the chicken broth, garlic seasoning and mushrooms. Using a wooden spoon, scrape the browned bits off the bottom of the pan. Cook for just 1 minute.
Add the pork tenderloin back to the pan and place in the oven for 15-25 minutes until pork is fully cooked (larger pieces will take a bit longer). Verify temp with meat thermometer. Pork should be 145 degrees F to be slightly pink, 160 for medium. Take it out at desired temp and let rest for 3 minutes before slicing. Note- If pork is cooked more than these recommended temperatures, it will be very dry and overdone.
Slice the pork and serve with the mushrooms and sauce. Serve hot with your favorite side dish.

- Serving Size: 5 oz. pork with 1 C mushrooms and is 1 Lean, 1 Green, 0 Healthy Fat and 2 Condiment options. Nutrition information below is for recipe made with pork tenderloin.

GARLIC SHRIMP & BROCCOLI

INGREDIENTS

- 4 teaspoons Roasted Garlic Oil (or fresh garlic and oil of your choice)
- 1 3/4 lbs wild caught shrimp, thawed and shells removed
- 2 C fresh broccoli florets
- 2 teaspoon Rockin' Ranch Seasoning (or tarragon, black pepper, salt, lemon, parsley, chives, garlic and onion)
- 1 teaspoon Garlic Gusto, Garlic & Spring Onion or Simply Brilliant Seasoning (or fresh garlic, lemon and onion)
- 1/3 C low sodium chicken broth
- 4 C alternative "noodles" of your choice (I used hearts of palm noodles in the image above)
- 2 Tablespoons butter

DIRECTION

Add oil to a large frying pan (with a lid) over medium high heat.
When oil is hot, add shrimp and cook for 1 minute on each side until slightly pink.

Add seasonings and broth to the shrimp. Stir to combine.

Add broccoli and place the cover on the pan. Bring to a boil and reduce heat to medium. Cook until broccoli is bright green (about 2 minutes). Remove the cover and add the butter. Stir to combine and then add the noodles. Toss the noodles in the liquid and cook until hot. Serve immediately.

- Serving Size: 7 oz. shrimp with 1/2 C broccoli and 1 C noodles and is 1 Lean, 3 Green, 2 Healthy Fat and 3 Condiment options.

MAKE CRISPY CROUTONS WITH THIS BISCUIT HACK

INGREDIENTS
- 1 packet Cheddar Herb Biscuits
- 2 Tablespoons water
- 1 Tablespoon lemon juice

DIRECTION
Pour contents of packet into a small bowl.

Add the water and juice and stir well with a small spatula.

Spray a medium sized, flat dish (or use a large bowl with a flat bottom) with nonstick cooking spray.

Pour the mixture into the dish and carefully spread into a thin layer. It should be about 1/4 inch thick.

Microwave on high for 2 minutes.

Carefully remove from the microwave, let cool and then break into pieces. Serve cool.

- Serving Size: 1/2 to 1 "biscuit" and is counted as one Meal Replacement (1/2 or 1 of the "5" in your 5 &1) Nutrition label from Cheddar Herb Biscuits and is 1 entire packet.

CHICKEN WITH GARLIC AND SPRING ONION CREAM

INGREDIENTS
- Nonstick cooking spray
- 1 1/2 lbs boneless, skinless chicken breasts, pounded to 3/8" thickness
- 1 teaspoons Dash of Desperation Seasoning (or nnatural sea salt and black pepper)

- 1 C low sodium chicken broth
- 2 teaspoons fresh lemon juice
- 1 Tablespoon (1 capful) Garlic and Spring Onion Seasoning (or fresh garlic, chives, salt, pepper and lemon)
- 4 Tablespoons lowfat cream cheese
- 2 Tablespoons butter
- fresh basil, parsley and/or lemon wedges for garnish if desired

DIRECTION

Pound chicken into 3/8" thickness. The easiest way to do this is to place one breast in a large plastic bag and hit with the back of a small frying pan. Be careful to do this on a cutting board, or other safe surface. You do not want to crack your countertops! Spray a large, nonstick pan with cooking spray and place the pan over medium-high heat.

Season each chicken breast with a pinch of Dash of Desperation Seasoning. When the pan is hot, place chicken in the pan.

Cook chicken for 5-7 minutes one one side then flip to the other side. Cook an additional 5 minutes more.

Add the broth, lemon juice and Garlic and Spring Onion to the pan. Stir well to combine. Using a spatula, scrape all the yummy brown bits off the bottom of the pan.

Let the mixture come to a simmer and continue to cook for 10-12 minutes until the sauce is reduced to only about 1/3 of a cup.

Add the cream cheese and butter to the pan and whisk to combine.

Remove from stove and sprinkle with fresh basil or other herbs and fresh lemon wedges or slices if desired. Serve hot with your favorite side dish.

- Serving Size: 6 oz. chicken with 1 T sauce and is 1 Lean, 1 Healthy Fat and 3 Condiment options.

CHICKEN WITH GARLIC AND SPRING ONION CREAM

INGREDIENTS

- cooking spray
- 1 1/2 lbs boneless, skinless chicken breasts, pounded to 3/8" thickness
- 1 teaspoons Dash of Desperation Seasoning (or nnatural sea salt and blk pacepper)
- 1 C low sodium chicken broth Nonstick
- 2 teaspoons fresh lemon juice
- 1 Tablespoon (1 capful) Garlic and Spring Onion Seasoning (or fresh garlic, chives, salt, pepper and lemon)
- 4 Tablespoons lowfat cream cheese
- 2 Tablespoons butter
- fresh basil, parsley and/or lemon wedges for garnish if desired

DIRECTION

Pound chicken into 3/8" thickness. The easiest way to do this is to place one breast in a large plastic bag and hit with the back of a small frying pan. Be careful to do this on a cutting board, or other safe surface. You do not want to crack your countertops!

Spray a large, nonstick pan with cooking spray and place the pan over medium-high heat.

Season each chicken breast with a pinch of Dash of Desperation Seasoning. When the pan is hot, place chicken in the pan.

Cook chicken for 5-7 minutes one one side then flip to the other side. Cook an additional 5 minutes more.

Add the broth, lemon juice and Garlic and Spring Onion to the pan. Stir well to combine. Using a spatula, scrape all the yummy brown bits off the bottom of the pan.

Let the mixture come to a simmer and continue to cook for 10-12 minutes until the sauce is reduced to only about 1/3 of a cup.

Add the cream cheese and butter to the pan and whisk to combine.

Remove from stove and sprinkle with fresh basil or other herbs and fresh lemon wedges or slices if desired. Serve hot with your favorite side dish.

- Serving Size: 6 oz. chicken with 1 T sauce and is 1 Lean, 1 Healthy Fat and 3 Condiment options.

CHEESY CHICKEN CAPRESE

INGREDIENTS
- 4 teaspoons Roasted Garlic Oil (or oil of your choice and fresh garlic)
- 1 1/2 lbs boneless, skinless chicken breasts, pounded to 3/8" thickness
- 2 teaspoons Tuscan Fantasty Seasoning (or garlic, red pepper, black pepper, parsley, onion, garlic powder)
- 1 C chopped tomatoes (can be fresh or canned and well drained)
- 8 Tablespoons (1/2 C) lowfat mozzarella cheese, shredded
- fresh basil for garnish if desired

DIRECTION
Preheat oven to 350 degrees.
Pound chicken into 3/8" thickness. The easiest way to do this is to place one breast in a large plastic bag and hit with the back of a small frying pan. Be careful to do this on a cutting board, or other safe surface. You do not want to crack your countertops! Add oil to a large, oven-safe frying pan (no plastic handles!) and place over medium-high heat.

Season each chicken breast with 1/2 teaspoon of Tuscan Fantasy seasoning. When the oil is hot, place chicken in the pan.

Cook chicken for 5-7 minutes one one side then flip to the other side. Cook an additional 5 minutes more.

Turn the stove off. Scoop 1/4 C tomatoes on to the top of each chicken breast.

Sprinkle 2 T mozzarella and an additional pinch of Tuscan Fantasy Seasoning over each chicken breast. Place in the oven for 7-10 minutes until chicken is fully cooked and cheese is melty. Verify temp with meat thermometer. Chicken should be 165 degrees F.

Remove from oven and sprinkle with fresh basil or other herbs if desired. Serve hot with your favorite side dish.

- Serving Size: 6 oz. chicken with 1/4 C tomatoes and 2 T cheese and is 1 Lean, 1/2 Green, 1 Healthy Fat and 3 Condiment options.

PAN SEARED BEEF TIPS AND MUSHROOMS

INGREDIENTS

- 1 1/2 lbs lean beef cut into 1" chunks (London broil, filet, strip stek, etc)
- 1/2 T Dasha of Desperation Seasoning (or salt, pepper and garlic)
- beef broth
- 11/2 teaspoons Garlic Gusto nonstick cooking spray
- 4 C mushrooms (either small, whole mushrooms or larger ones cut into quarters)
- 1 C low sodium or Garlic & Spring Onion Seasoning (or fresh garlic, parsley and onion)

DIRECTION

Add beef to a bowl and sprinkle with seasoning. Toss to coat evenly.

Place a well-seasoned cast iron pan on the stove over high heat. If you do not have one, use a nonstick skillet and spray with nonstick spray.

Add the beef to the pan in a single layer. Let it cook for 5-7 minutes until a rich, browned crust forms on the meat. Flip the meat to the other side and repeat the process to brown on the other side.

Remove the meat from the pan and place in a bowl.
Cover with a clean kitchen towel to keep warm.
Turn the heat to medium high and pour in the
broth. Use a wooden spoon to scrape all the
browned bits off the bottom of the pan. Add the
Garlic Gusto seasoning and the mushrooms and let
the mixture simmer until it is reduced by half.
Add the beef back to the pan and toss to coat in the
sauce. Serve hot.

- Serving Size: 5 oz. beef with 1 C mushrooms
  and 2 T sauce and is 1 Lean, 1 Green, 0
  Healthy Fat and 2 Condiment options.

TURMERIC GINGER SPICED CAULIFLOWER

INGREDIENTS

- 4 C cauliflower florets, larger sized
- 2 C carrots or yellow/orange/red bell pepper cut into strips
- 4 teaspoons oil*
- 1/2 teaspoons Dash of Desperation or Salt and pepper to taste
- 1/4 C low sodium chicken broth
- 1 teaspoons Garlic Gusto Seasoning (or fresh garlic, parsley and lemon spritz)
- 1/2 teaspoons Spices of India (or curry powder)

DIRECTION

Set oven to broil and place rack on the second shelf down in the oven. Veggies should cook 6-8" away from heat source if possible.

Toss vegetables with oil (* if you do not have room for a Healthy Fat in your meal, substitute 1/4 C of chicken broth instead) and season with Dash of Desperation Seasoning.
Spread veggie mixture evenly on a cookie sheet and broil for 12-15 minutes until slightly charred. At the

6 minute mark, using tongs or a spatula turn the veggies over to promote browning on all sides. Place a large, nonstick pan over medium high heat on the stovetop. When veggies have finished broiling, add broth and Garlic Gusto to the pan. Once bubbling, add veggies and cook for 5 minutes until liquid has evaporated.

Sprinkle with Spices of India and toss to coat. Cook one-2 additional minutes to toast the spices and then serve hot. Season with additional salt and pepper if desired.

- Serving Size: 1 C vegetable mixture (using peppers) and is 0 Lean, 2 Green, 0-1 Healthy Fat and 1 Condiment options. Nutrition information below is for one serving with cauliflower and orange peppers cooked in broth, not oil. If using oil, add 1 healthy fat and 40 calories.

MIDDLE EASTERN MEATBALLS WITH DILL SAUCE

INGREDIENTS

- 1 1/2 lbs lean ground beef (or ground chicken, lamb, turkey or pork or a combination)
- 2 teaspoons Spices of India (or curry powder)
- 1/4 teaspoon Sinful Cinnamon or ground cinnamon & a pinch of nutmeg
- Salt and pepper to taste
- 1/2 C plain, lowfat Greek yogurt
- 11/2 teaspoons Citrus Dill or fresh dill, onion, chives and lemon)

DIRECTION

Add seasoning to beef and mix well to combine. Divide mixture into 20 even portions and roll into balls.
Place a nonstick pan over medium high heat and add the meatballs once pan has come to temperature.
Cook for 15-20 minutes, turning meatballs every 2-3 minutes so they brown equally on all sides.

While beef is cooking, make the sauce by combining the yogurt and Citrus Dill seasoning together. Stir well & keep in fridge until ready to eat.
When meatballs are finished (internal temperature of 160 F) place on a plate and serve hot with sauce.

- Serving Size: 5 oz. ground beef with 1 T sauce and is 1 Lean, 0 Green, 0 Healthy Fat and 2 Condiment options. Nutrition information below is for one serving with ground beef and 1 T sauce.

CREAMY SKILLET CHICKEN AND ASPARAGUS

INGREDIENTS
- 4 teaspoons Roasted Garlic Oil (or oil of your choice and fresh garlic)
- 1 3/4 lbs boneless, skinless chicken breast, cut into 1" chunks
- 1/2 C low sodium chicken broth
- 1 Tablespoon (one capful) Garlic and Spring Onion or Garlic Gusto Seasoning or fresh chopped garlic, parsley and chives
- 8 T (4 oz or half an 8 oz block) light cream cheese
- 4 C fresh asparagus, cut into 2" pieces
- Pinch Dash of Desperation Seasoning (or salt and pepper and garlic)

DIRECTION
Add oil to a large skillet and heat over medium high heat.

When hot, add chicken breasts and cook for 7-10 minutes, stirring occasionally. The chicken should be slightly browned.

Pour the broth into the pan and, using a spatula, scrape all the browned bits (fond) off the bottom of the pan.

Add garlic seasoning, cream cheese and asparagus. Turn the heat to high.

Stir the ingredients continually, allowing the cream cheese to melt evenly into the sauce. Bring to a boil and simmer until a thick, rich sauce has formed. Divide into 4 equal portions, sprinkle with a little Dash of Desperation and serve hot.

- Serving Size: (1/4 of this dish) is approximately 6 oz. chicken with 2 T sauce and 1 C asparagus and is 1 Leaner, 2 Green, 1 Healthy Fat and 3 Condiment options.

SEARED MAHI MAHI WITH LEMON BASIL BUTTER

INGREDIENTS
- 4 Tablespoons butter
- 1 Tablespoon Garlic and Spring Onion or Garlic Gusto Seasoning or fresh chopped garlic, parsley and chives
- 2 Tablespoons fresh chopped basil leaves
- 1 Tablespoon fresh squeezed lemon juice
- Nonstick cooking spray
- 2 pounds fresh, wild caught Mahi Mahi filets (or other flaky white fish, shrimp or thinly sliced chicken)
- Pinch Dash of Desperation Seasoning (or salt and pepper and garlic)

DIRECTION
Add butter to a small sauce pot and melt over low heat. Add garlic seasoning, basil and lemon. Stir to combine. Set aside and keep warm (or reheat when fish is almost fully cooked.)
Spray a large, nonstick frying pan with nonstick cooking spray and heat over medium-high. (Redundant, yes, but fish is so delicate you just want to make sure. You could use a little butter or

oil here instead if not on 5&1 or on a fat-restricted program.)

Sprinkle the fish with Dash of Desperation.

When pan is hot add the fish and let it cook for 2-3 minutes on each side until opaque and fully cooked. Be sure not to overcook the fish as it will be dry and chewy.

Gently remove the fish from the pan and drizzle with warm hot, melted butter. Serve warm with your favorite side dish. Makes about 4 servings.

- Serving Size: is 7 ounces of fish with 1 Tablespoon of butter and is 1 Leanest, 3 Condiment and 2 Healthy Fat options.

TOASTED SESAME GINGER CHICKEN

INGREDIENTS

- 4 teaspoons Valencia Orange Oil or oil of your choice and orange zest
- 1 1/2 lbs boneless, skinless chicken breast
- 1 Tablespoon Toasted Sesame Ginger Seasoning (or toasted sesame seeds, garlic, onion powder, red pepper, ground ginger, salt, pepper and lemon)

DIRECTION

Place chicken breasts on a clean, dry cutting board. Using a meat mallet or back side of a frying pan, gently flatten the chicken breasts to appprox. 3/8" thickness.

Sprinkle with seasoning.

Heat Valencia Orange Oil in a large, nonstick frying pan over medium - high heat.

Add chicken and cook for 7-8 minutes on one side, until a lovely crust has formed- it will be slightly brown.

Gently flip chicken and cook on the other side for an additional 5-6 minutes until chicken is fully cooked.

Serve warm with your favorite side dish, or chilled over salad. Makes about 4 servings.

- Serving Size: is 6 ounces of chicken and is 1 Lean, 1 Condiment and 1 Healthy Fat option.

TENDER AND TASTY FISH TACOS

INGREDIENTS

- 1 3/4 lbs cod or haddock (wild caught)
- 1 capful (1 Tablespoon) Southwestern Seasoning or Phoenix Sunrise Seasoning or cumin, cilantro, garlic, onion, red pepper,

paprika, parsley, salt & pepper (or low sodium taco seasoning)
- 4 teaspoons Roasted Garlic Oil or oil of your choice and fresh garlic
- your favorite taco condiments

DIRECTION

Pat fish dry and cut into 1" chunks

Sprinkle seasoning over fish and toss to coat.

Heat Roasted Garlic Oil in a large, nonstick frying pan over medium - high heat.

Add fish and cook for 10 - 12 minutes, until fish is opaque and breaks apart into flakes. Be careful not to overcook or the fish will be dry and chewy.

Serve hot with your favorite condiments.

Makes about 4 servings.

- Serving Size: is 7 ounces of fish. Nutrition information and counts below is for fish & seasoning only. For condiments, please adjust counts and calories accordingly.

SAUSAGE STUFFED MUSHROOMS - A LBD LG RECIPE

INGREDIENTS
- 4 large portobello mushrooms (caps and stems)
- 1 1/2 pounds lean Italian sausage (85-94% lean)
- 1 capful (1 Tablespoon) Garlic & Spring Onion Seasoning or Garlic Gusto Seasoning or chopped garlic, chopped chives, garlic powder, onion powder, salt and pepper to taste

DIRECTION
Preheat oven to 350 degrees.
Gently remove the mushroom stems & wash both the caps and stems
Chop the stems into small pieces and place in a bowl. Add the meat and seasoning to the bowl and using your hands, combine all ingredients well.
Place the mushroom caps smooth side down on a large cookie sheet or baking tray.
Divide the meat mixture into 4 equal parts and gently press one portion into each mushroom cap.
Bake for approximately 25 minutes & serve hot with your favorite side dishes.

Makes about 4 servings.
- Serving : is 5 ounces of meat and 1 cup of mushrooms per portion.

SMOKY SHRIMP CHIPOTLE

INGREDIENTS
- 4 teaspoons Roasted Garlic Oil or oil of your choice and fresh garlic
- 1 C chopped chives or scallions (greens only)
- 2 lbs wild caught, raw shrimp, shelled, deveined & tails removed
- 1 can (~16 oz) diced tomatoes (unflavored, no sugar added)
- 1 capful (1 Tablespoon) Cinnamon Chipotle or a small amount of chipotle pepper, cinnamon, salt and pepper to taste
- 4 lime wedges (optional)
- 4 T fresh cilantro (optional)

DIRECTION
Heat oil in a medium sized frying pan over medium high heat.

Add the scallions and cook for one minute, until slightly wilted and glistening.

Add the shrimp and cook for 1 minute on each side.

Add the tomatoes and Cinnamon Chipotle seasoning. Cook an additional 3-5 minutes, stirring occasionally, until the tomatoes are hot and shrimp is opaque & fully cooked. Be careful not to overcook as it will make the shrimp tough and dry.

Sprinkle with cilantro if desired and spritz with a wedge of lime (or serve the lime wedge on the plate for a pretty and functional garnish.

Serve warm.

Makes about 4 servings.

- Serving Size: is 7 ounces of shrimp and 1/4 of the sauce mixture. Nutritional information and counts below include cilantro and lime (1.5 condiments for both)

LOW CARB SLOPPY JOES

INGREDIENTS

- 1 1/2 pounds lean ground beef
- 1/2 C diced green bell pepper
- 2 Tablespoons tomato paste
- 1 teaspoon (one packet) powdered stevia
- 1 Tablespoon yellow mustard
- 1Tablespoon (one Capful) Garlic & Spring Onion Seasoning or salt, pepper, crushed garlic, garlic powder and onion to taste
- 1/2 Tablespoon Cinnamon Chipotle Seasoning or ground cinnamon, chipotle paste and garlic
- 1Tablespoon ed wine vinegar
- 1 C low sodium beef broth
- Dash of Desperation or Salt and Pepper to taste

DIRECTION

Place the ground beef in a frying pan and place on the stove over medium heat. Break up the larger pieces of meat as it is cooking.

Let the meat cook for about 7 minutes and then add the remaining ingredients (EXCEPT the broth) and stir to combine. Once mixed, add the water and turn up the heat to medium high.

Once the liquid is boiling, reduce the heat to low and let it simmer, uncovered for about 10-15 minutes until the liquid is somewhat reduced & you have a lovely sauce.

Serve hot & enjoy!

- Serving Size: is 5 ounces of ground beef and pepper mixture & approx 1 T sauce. Nutrition Information is for beef mixture only.

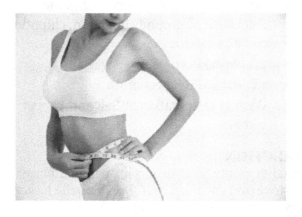

PAN SEARED BALSAMIC CHICKEN AND VEGETABLES

INGREDIENTS

- 1 1/2 pounds boneless, skinless chicken thighs
- 1Tablespoon (one Capful) Tuscan Fantasy Seasoning or salt, pepper, garlic, red pepper, parsley, garlic powder and onion to taste
- 4Tablespoon Balsamic Mosto Cotto or balsamic reduction
- 1Tablespoon Dijon Mustard
- 2 C cherry or grape tomatoes, halved
- 2 C zucchini sliced into 3/8" slices (try to have the zucchini around 1" in diameter-smaller ones cook faster and have less seeds)
- 1/3 C water

DIRECTION

Whisk together balsamic, mustard and seasoning in a bowl large enough to hold the chicken.
Add the chicken and toss to coat. Place in the refrigerator for 20 minutes, up to 8 hours to marinade.
When ready to cook, preheat oven to 425 degrees.

Place a well-seasoned cast iron skillet (large enough to hold all the chicken without crowding) over medium-high heat.

Shake off the excess marinade (reserving it in the bowl for later) and place the chicken in the pan.

Cook until seared and slightly browned, about 5 minutes. Flip chicken and cook an additional 5 minutes on the other side.While chicken is cooking, prepare the vegetables.

Add water to remaining marinade in the bowl and whisk to combine.

Scatter the vegetables around the pan. Season with a pinch of salt and pepper (or   Dash of Desperation for additional flavor).

Pour the marinade mixture over the veggies & chicken. Toss to combine together. Place in the preheated oven for 15 minutes additional.

Remove from oven and serve hot.

- Serving Size: is 5 ounces of chicken, 1 C of vegetables and 2 T sauce.

FRESH LIME CREMA

INGREDIENTS
- Cup sour cream
- 1teaspoon (one Capful) Dash of Desperation Seasoning or salt, pepper, garlic and onion to taste
- zest from one lime
- juice from one lime
- 1/4 C fresh cilantro, finely shredded if desired

DIRECTION
Place all ingredients in a mixing bowl and stir vigorously to combine.
Let rest for 15 minutes before serving to allow flavors to develop. May be stored in an airtight container, refrigerated for up to one week.
- Serving Size: is 1 Tablespoon of crema.

FRESH PICO DE GALLO

INGREDIENTS

- 1 C diced tomatoes (fresh or canned and well drained)
- 1/4 C (4 Tablespoons) fresh onion, finely chopped
- 1teaspoon Dash of Desperation Seasoning or salt, pepper, garlic and onion to taste
- 2 T finely chopped cilantro
- juice of one fresh lime

DIRECTION

Place all ingredients in a bowl and toss gently to combine.

For best flavor, let sit for 15 minutes before serving. May make ahead of time and store in an airtight container in the refrigerator for up to 1 week.

- Serving Size: is either 1/2 C (1 Green Serving) or 1 Tablespoon (1 Condiment Serving) Nutrition information below is for 1/2 C (8 Tablespoons)

TEX-MEX SEARED SALMON

INGREDIENTS

- 1 1/2 pounds wild caught salmon filet (will cook best if you have it at room temp)
- 1Tablespoon (one Capful) Phoenix Sunrise Seasoning or salt, pepper, garlic, cumin, paprika, cayenne and onion to taste

DIRECTION

Preheat nonstick pan over high heat for 1 minute. While heating, sprinkle seasoning over the salmon (NOT on the skin side)

Reduce heat to medium high.

Place the fish, seasoning side down in the pan and let it cook for 4-6 minutes depending on thickness. You'll know it's ready to flip when a "crust" has formed from the seasoning and the fish releases from the pan easily.

Reduce heat to medium low. Flip the fish over to skin side down and cook an additional 4-6 minutes. (Less for medium/rare and more for well done.) The best method to check for doneness is to use a meat thermometer. We cook to 130 degrees and then let it rest for 5 minutes for slightly pink and not overcooked.

Remove from heat and serve. Fish should slide right off the skin and on to the plate.

- Serving Size: is 5 ounces of salmon

CHARRED SIRLOIN WITH CREAMY HORSERADISH SAUCE

INGREDIENTS
- 1 1/2 pounds sirloin steaks, trimmed & visible fat removed
- 1/2 capful (1/2 Tablesoon) Dash of Desperation Seasoning or salt, pepper, garlic and onion to taste
- 6 Tablespoons lowfat sour cream
- 1-3 T horseradish (from the jar)

DIRECTION
Preheat grill to medium-high heat.
the steak on both sides with Dash of Desperation Seasoning
Place on the grill and cook for 5-7 minutes on each side, depending on how thick the steak is and the way you like your meat cooked. You'll leave it on less for rare and more for medium-well. The BEST way to cook the steak is by using a meat thermometer.
While meat is cooking, make the sauce by combining together the sour cream and

horseradish. Add water, one Tablespoon at a time to thin the mixture to make a sauce. Set aside when done.

When the meat is finished cooking, let it rest on a cutting board for 5 minutes, then slice thin.

- Serve drizzled with 1-2 T of sauce.
- Serving Size: is 5 ounces of sliced steak and 1-2 T Sauce (Sauce is 1 Condiment per Tablespoon) This recipe serves approximately 4. Nutrition information is calculated with 5 oz steak and 1 T sauce. Zucchini noodle counts not included.

ROASTED GARLIC ZOODLES

INGREDIENTS
- 1Tablespoon Roasted Garlic Oil) or other fat of your choice*
- 6 Cups zucchini noodles
- 1/2 capful (1/2 Tablesoon) Garlic and Spring Onion Seasoning or Garlic Gusto Seasoning) or fresh chopped garlic, salt and pepper
- Pinch of salt and pepper or Dash of Desperation Seasoning to taste

DIRECTION
Add the oil / spray to a larger sized frying pan and heat over medium-high heat.
Add the zucchini noodles to the pan and sprinkle with seasoning.
Cook for just 2-3 minutes, tossing occasionally with a pair of tongs.
Season with a pinch of salt and pepper (or Dash of Desperation Seasoning for more pop!) and serve hot.
*You may make a no-fat version of this recipe simply by using nonstick cooking spray instead of oil. Nutrition information is calculated using oil.
- Serving Size: is 1 1/2 Cups cooked, seasoned zoodles. This recipe serves approximately 4.

HEAVENLY GREEN BEANS AND GARLIC

INGREDIENTS

- 1 1/2 pounds green beans (about 4 cups) ends trimmed
- 1/2 capful (1/2 Tablesoon) Garlic and Spring Onion Seasoning or Garlic Gusto Seasoning) or fresh chopped garlic, salt and pepper
- 1Tablespoon Roasted Garlic Oil) or other fat of your choice*
- 4 Tablespoons freshly grated Parmesan cheese

DIRECTION

Place green beans in a pot with a lid and add 1" of water to the bottom.

Sprinkle seasoning over the top of the beans, trying to keep most of the seasoning on the beans and out of the water.

Place the covered pot on the stove over high heat. Bring water to a boil and let the beans steam for 5-7 minutes, until bright green and crisp tender. Be careful not to over cook.

Carefully drain all the water out of the pot.

Drizzle with Roasted Garlic Oil and a pinch of salt and pepper (or Dash of Desperation Seasoning for more pop!) Sprinkle with cheese and serve hot.

- Serving Size: is 1 C cooked, seasoned green beans. This recipe serves approximately 4.

LOW CARB TACO BOWLS

INGREDIENTS
- 1 large head cauliflower, steamed until soft or frozen ready-to-cook cauliflower rice
- 1 1/2 pounds lean ground beef
- 1-2 capfuls Phoenix Sunrise or Southwestern Seasoning (or a combination of both!) or low salt taco seasoning
- 2 C canned, diced tomatoes (no sugar added, no flavor added)
- Your favorite approved condiments*.

DIRECTION
Place a large frying pan over medium high heat. Add ground beef to a large (preferably nonstick) pan and saute for 8-12 minutes until slightly browned. Break up the larger chunks into smaller pieces using a spatula or a chopping tool.
Add tomatoes and seasoning. Stir to combine. Reduce the heat to low and allow the mixture to

cook for 5 minutes, until the liquid is reduced by 1/2 and nice & thick.

While the meat is cooking, use a food processor or chopping tool to chop steamed cauliflower up into rice-sized bits. If using ready-to-cook cauli rice, prepare it according to package DIRECTION.

Place 1/2 C cauliflower rice into a bowl and top with 1/4 of the meat mixture. Top with your favorite condiments* and serve hot.

- Serving Size: is 1/4 of the beef mixture and 1/2 C of cauliflower rice. This recipe as prepared serves 4 people. Nutrition information is for beef/tomato mixture and rice only. Please adjust for condiments.

Cooking Basics Checklist

Prepare

- ☐ Read the recipe, do any preheating
- ☐ Get all the ingredients and cooking gear out
- ☐ Prepare all ingredients per the instructions

Work safely

- ☐ Position pot/pan handles to prevent accidents
- ☐ Place a shelf liner or damp kitchen towel under cutting boards to prevent slipping
- ☐ Wash any items immediately after touching raw meat to prevent cross-contamination

Work clean

- ☐ Keep a kitchen towel close to wipe down
- ☐ Wipe cutting boards as you go
- ☐ Keep trashcan or another disposal nearby

Learn basic prep and cooking skills

- ☐ Chop an onion
- ☐ Hard- or soft-boil an egg
- ☐ Poach an egg
- ☐ Cook pasta and rice
- ☐ Melt chocolate
- ☐ Make a scrambled egg or an omelet
- ☐ Bake a potato
- ☐ Stuff and roast a chicken (or turkey)
- ☐ Make gravy
- ☐ Make stock
- ☐ Separate an egg
- ☐ Knead dough
- ☐ Crush and chop garlic
- ☐ Prepare peppers
- ☐ Brown meat
- ☐ Cook a perfect steak
- ☐ Make salad dressing
- ☐ Make batter
- ☐ Rub flour and butter
- ☐ Line a cake tin
- ☐ Make tomato sauce
- ☐ Pit an avocado
- ☐ Whip cream
- ☐ Segment an orange

Master key cooking methods

- ☐ Braising
- ☐ Roasting
- ☐ Boiling
- ☐ Baking
- ☐ Browning
- ☐ Searing
- ☐ Grilling
- ☐ Frying
- ☐ Basting
- ☐ Broiling

Cooking Basics Checklist

Prepare
- ☐ Read the recipe, do any preheating
- ☐ Get all the ingredients and cooking gear out
- ☐ Prepare all ingredients per the instructions

Work safely
- ☐ Position pot/pan handles to prevent accidents
- ☐ Place a shelf liner or damp kitchen towel under cutting boards to prevent slipping
- ☐ Wash any items immediately after touching raw meat to prevent cross-contamination

Work clean
- ☐ Keep a kitchen towel close to wipe down
- ☐ Wipe cutting boards as you go
- ☐ Keep trashcan or another disposal nearby

Learn basic prep and cooking skills
- ☐ Chop an onion
- ☐ Hard- or soft-boil an egg
- ☐ Poach an egg
- ☐ Cook pasta and rice
- ☐ Melt chocolate
- ☐ Make a scrambled egg or an omelet
- ☐ Bake a potato
- ☐ Stuff and roast a chicken (or turkey)
- ☐ Make gravy
- ☐ Make stock
- ☐ Separate an egg
- ☐ Knead dough
- ☐ Crush and chop garlic
- ☐ Prepare peppers
- ☐ Brown meat
- ☐ Cook a perfect steak
- ☐ Make salad dressing
- ☐ Make batter
- ☐ Rub flour and butter
- ☐ Line a cake tin
- ☐ Make tomato sauce
- ☐ Pit an avocado
- ☐ Whip cream
- ☐ Segment an orange

Master key cooking methods
- ☐ Braising
- ☐ Roasting
- ☐ Boiling
- ☐ Baking
- ☐ Browning
- ☐ Searing
- ☐ Grilling
- ☐ Frying
- ☐ Basting
- ☐ Broiling

METABOLIC DIET

Cooking Basics Checklist

Prepare
- [ ] Read the recipe, do any preheating
- [ ] Get all the ingredients and cooking gear out
- [ ] Prepare all ingredients per the instructions

Work safely
- [ ] Position pot/pan handles to prevent accidents
- [ ] Place a shelf liner or damp kitchen towel under cutting boards to prevent slipping
- [ ] Wash any items immediately after touching raw meat to prevent cross-contamination

Work clean
- [ ] Keep a kitchen towel close to wipe down
- [ ] Wipe cutting boards as you go
- [ ] Keep trashcan or another disposal nearby

Learn basic prep and cooking skills
- [ ] Chop an onion
- [ ] Hard- or soft-boil an egg
- [ ] Poach an egg
- [ ] Cook pasta and rice
- [ ] Melt chocolate
- [ ] Make a scrambled egg or an omelet
- [ ] Bake a potato
- [ ] Stuff and roast a chicken (or turkey)
- [ ] Make gravy
- [ ] Make stock
- [ ] Separate an egg
- [ ] Knead dough
- [ ] Crush and chop garlic
- [ ] Prepare peppers
- [ ] Brown meat
- [ ] Cook a perfect steak
- [ ] Make salad dressing
- [ ] Make batter
- [ ] Rub flour and butter
- [ ] Line a cake tin
- [ ] Make tomato sauce
- [ ] Pit an avocado
- [ ] Whip cream
- [ ] Segment an orange

Master key cooking methods
- [ ] Braising
- [ ] Roasting
- [ ] Boiling
- [ ] Baking
- [ ] Browning
- [ ] Searing
- [ ] Grilling
- [ ] Frying
- [ ] Basting
- [ ] Broiling

CPSIA information can be obtained
at www.ICGtesting.com
Printed in the USA
BVHW041509110321
602278BV00012B/1108

9 781801 470674